The  e
Diet Handbook

Walkthrough, 200+ Foods to Eat & Avoid, 21 Delicious Starter Recipes, Index of Medical Condition Relationships Such as Kidney Stones, and More!

by

ELIZABETH GRAY

Copyright © 2018 by Elizabeth Gray

All rights reserved. This book or any portion thereof
may not be reproduced or used in any manner whatsoever
without the express written permission of the publisher
except for the use of brief quotations in a book review.
Printed in the United States of America
First Printing, 2018

ISBN-13:
978-1719543231
ISBN-10:
1719543232

Elizabeth Gray Publishing
18 Key Street
Millis, MA 02054

Your diet is a bank account. Good food choices are good investments.

~ BETHENNY FRANKEL

DISCLAIMER

The information in this book does not contain medical professional advice. Individuals requiring such services should consult a competent medical professional. The author makes no representations about the suitability of the information contained in this book for any purpose. This material is provided "as is" and this publication is for informational purposes only.

TABLE OF CONTENTS

Introduction 1

What is Oxalate Anyway? 4

Measuring the Oxalate Level 6

Help in Preventing Kidney Stones 8

Low Oxalate Foods May Help Other Health Conditions 11

Listing of Foods with Oxalate Levels 14

Notes on Some Favorite Foods 27

Other Tips for a Low Oxalate Diet 30

Low Oxalate Help at Meals 33

Recipes 36

    Breakfast 39

    Lunch 44

    Dinner 49

    Desserts 54

Last Word on a Low Oxalate Diet 60

Can I Ask You a Favor? 61

INTRODUCTION

You may have already heard of the low oxalate diet. Your doctor may have suggested you try it for a number of health issues with the most common condition being kidney stones. A low oxalate diet often is beneficial for other health concerns too…such as children with autism or adults with fibromyalgia. Or if your doctor just can't figure out where your joint aches and pains are coming from, they may suggest you give this diet a try to see if your symptoms improve.

Thus, oxalates have gained attention in health news recently and a growing number of people are reducing the amount of oxalate in their diet for a number of various health reasons.

I have written this book mainly because many of my friends have gotten kidney stones. They were surprised to get the kidney stones in the first place, and then their physicians recommend a low oxalate diet. They consider themselves pretty savvy when it comes to eating good food yet they never heard of a low oxalate diet.

It's not like a diet where you give up one food group entirely such as giving up carbohydrates to lose weight. They were given a list of foods with their oxalate content described as high, moderate, and low. And guess what? Since they eat healthy food most of the time, they were shocked when their physicians said stay away from spinach! Now, the diet is still controversial and there are many differences what oxalate levels foods should go into…but all the diet lists (and physicians) agree. Spinach is a very high oxalate food!

Many people are confused from this alone. And rightly they should be. We were all told spinach was good for your body for many years. My hope for this book is to demystify the low oxalate diet which will become even more popular. As of this writing, there are many variations in reported amounts of oxalates in food. New methods of measure often mean established lists of food are not right causing much confusion. Oxalate content varies not only for food but can also vary depending on what type of cooking or processing method is used, the soil content, the time of harvest, and whether the food is fresh or canned.

I am trying a low oxalate diet as I do not want to experience a kidney stones as unfortunately, my sister has them many times. In fact, kidney stones are on the rise and doctors are recommending a low oxalate diet more and more to prevent them. Frankly, we do not know what is causing this rise. The rise may be explained for many reasons and research is still unclear why this is happening. But having kidney stones is no laughing matter. Kidney stones are not the most serious health problem but passing one can be one of the most painful activities for humans. In fact, women who have given birth to children have often compared passing a kidney stone to labor!

This book will help you understand what oxalate is and why you may consider a low oxalate diet whether it's to get less kidney stones or minimize other symptoms for another medical issue. I am not a medical professional so I stress that you speak to your physician about your unique medical situation.

To keep track of low oxalate foods may seem overwhelming at first especially since the oxalate content of foods is not listed on food labels. This book strives to make you an intelligent consumer which will then enable you to ask your doctor intelligent questions. And back to spinach…there are a lot of healthy options out there to replace it! The vegetables just aren't as popular and we just don't know much about them yet. So don't walk out depressed from your doctor's office (many types of fruit are often high oxalate too and, oh, chocolate too). But hopefully, you can replace these foods, grow to not miss them. After all, isn't it worth it to give up some foods if it makes you feel much better?

What is Oxalate Anyway?

Forgive me for getting scientific for a moment.

According to Merriam Webster, "oxalate is a salt or ester of oxalic acid." (If you don't know the definition of ester, like I didn't (!), it's any of a class of often fragrant organic compounds that can be represented by the formula RCOOR' and that are usually formed by the reaction between an acid and an alcohol with elimination of water.)

And the definition of oxalic acid is "a poisonous strong acid $(COOH)_2$ or $H_2C_2O_4$ that occurs in various plants (such as spinach) as oxalates and is used especially as a bleaching or cleaning agent and as a chemical intermediate."

Or to put it simply and for our purposes, just remember, an oxalate is a naturally occurring molecule found in plants and humans. It is not a required nutrient for people. Our bodies make oxalate on their own. But recent studies cannot find evidence that oxalate has a beneficial reason at all in humans. It's thought to be a useless end product of carbohydrate metabolism and is usually excreted through the stool with no problems.

In plants, oxalate helps to get rid of extra calcium by "binding" with it. In humans, it may be nondigestive but feeds good bacteria to the gut. Thus, oxalate passes through the intestines, and leaves the body if it's combined with calcium, and excreted in the stool. However, by getting too much oxalate, it can get trapped in the kidney, leading to kidney stones.

Kidney stones are fortunately easy to diagnose. But other strange symptoms can develop without getting kidney stones in your body. Excessive amounts of oxalates can lead to oxidative damage and the depletion of a substance called glutathione. Another problem with excess oxalates, they can bind to other minerals and prevent the body from absorbing some important ones.

This can also cause other health problems that are difficult to treat. Some of them include: burning urination, leaky gut, vulvodynia, chronic fatigue, cystic fibrosis, autism, fibromyalgia, joint pain (arthritis), and even insomnia!

If you have one of these conditions, you may have an oxalate sensitivity. If you do not have enough healthy bacteria to break down oxalates before they can reach other parts of your body, you may benefit from a low oxalate diet.

Measuring the Oxalate Level

As mentioned, oxalate is primarily found in plants. So the listing of whether a food is high, moderate, or low in oxalate can be very confusing. For the measuring of oxalate levels often depends on when the food is harvested, where the food is grown, and how its oxalate level was tested.

But we may ask ourselves, "Why does nature put oxalate in plants anyway (especially spinach!)." According to studies, plants use oxalate to protect themselves from infection and from being eaten. Oxalate taste good to bugs that may eat the plants. They'll eat the oxalate and not the plants themselves. They will leave the plants alone.

But this can be dangerous for larger species. This is why certain plants are dangerous to our pets. The pet poison helpline says many common indoor and outdoor plants, contain insoluble calcium oxalate crystals. Examples include Dieffenbachia, Calla lily, Arrowhead, Dumbcane, PeaceLily, Philodendron, Pothos, Umbrella Plant, Elephant's Ear, Chinese Evergreen, and Schefflera. Chewing or biting into these plants will release the crystals causing tissue penetration and irritation to the mouth and GI tract. VERY rarely, swelling of the upper airway occurs, making it difficult to breathe. Insoluble calcium oxalate-containing plants have a different mechanism of toxicity than soluble oxalate-containing plants (e.g., star fruit, rhubarb, shamrock).

Most of the oxalate foods we eat are soluble or a simple way to put it, able to dissolve in water. These are thus more easily absorbed and usually excreted through the stool or urine. But anyone trying to lower oxalates in a diet should know a food's level and that's where a low oxalate diet comes in.
For a leafy vegetables such as spinach are known to contain moderate amounts of soluble and insoluble oxalates.

So soluble forms can dissolve completely in liquid meaning they can pass though the body quite easily. But insoluble forms can lodge in tissues and cause lots of inflammation. Obviously, this is a complex topic but let me try to put it in simple language. Think of it this way. Soluble means moveable. And insoluble means immobile. It is difficult for insoluble oxalate to be absorbed by the body but easy for them to leave in the stool.

But also remember, this is only true in healthy people. Oxalates should be absorbed by the body or eliminated. But often oxalates are leading to kidney stones and other health problems. So they may not be so good for you.

Let's investigate what we can do to prevent health issues like kidney stones and why we may want to consider a low oxalate diet.

Help in Preventing Kidney Stones

By now you know that your daily intake of calcium is important. You should make sure you're getting enough calcium especially on a low oxalate diet. (And no, I do not work for the dairy industry. Calcium can be found in other food groups as well other than dairy.)

Let me explain using kidney stones as an example. If there is enough calcium in your diet, the calcium binds to oxalate. Many people are afraid to eat calcium rich foods because of the name "calcium oxalate stones". These are the most common type of kidney stones. Roughly, calcium oxalate stones are 80% of the stones tested with about one million people developing kidney stones. They are most likely to affect adults between the ages of 20 through 40.

According to research, diets that are low in calcium can raise urine oxalate levels. Higher calcium levels can inhibit this, the intestinal oxalate absorption. For on its way through the intestines, oxalate can bind with calcium and be safely be excreted through the stool. Small kidney stones pass through the urinary tract with no pain. It's when high levels of oxalate continuously pass through the kidneys, larger kidney stones develop. Thus, the name calcium oxalate kidney stones. In fact, a low oxalate diet is often called the kidney stone diet.

People, known as stone formers, should increase not decrease their amount of calcium. Because the calcium binds oxalate in the intestines, a diet rich in calcium helps reduce the amount of oxalate being absorbed by the body, so stones are less likely to form. Also, eating foods high in calcium along with foods that are high in oxalate reduces your risk to forming calcium oxalate kidney stones. Therefore, it's good to be aware of how many oxalates you are eating. Consider meeting with a registered dietician to help you figure this out.

But first find out what type of stones you have from your physician. It may be hard to believe, but many people do not know this! They probable are so happy to get rid of their stone and of the pain. Not all stones are created equal. In addition to the calcium oxalate stones mentioned above, another common type is uric acid stones. This type of stone develops when your urine is too acidic.

A diet rich in purines can increase the acidic level. Simply put, purine is a colorless substance found in fish, shellfish, and meats. For these, you should concentrate mainly on vegetables and fruits.

Struvite stones are found mostly in women with urinary tract infections. They result from a kidney infection and should be treated. Finally, cysteine stones are very rare. They occur in adults who have the genetic disorder, cystinuria. Cystine, an acid that occurs naturally in the body, leaks from the kidneys into the urine.

Your doctor may prescribe a medication too with stones, known as an alpha blocker, which can relax the muscles in your ureter, helping you to pass a stone more easily and less painfully. The type of medication will depend on what type of kidney stones you have.

Low Oxalate Foods May Help Other Health Conditions

Mainstream medicine has usually proclaimed that you don't have to worry about going on a low oxalate diet unless you develop kidney stones. But it has often been found that going on a low oxalate diet can help in other health situations too in people who've no history of kidney stones. Next we examine some of these.

Following a low oxalate diet may help in conditions such as autism, vulvodynia, vaginodynia, chronic fatigue, fibromyalgia and leaky gut.

Following a low oxalate diet can help in the overall healing process for autism. Of course, the diet isn't the only solution but it can help. Parents of an autistic child have seen verbal and social skills improve when children go on the diet. Improvements with urinary urgency, constipation, and diarrhea are often reported. Find a doctor who is a specialist in this area and see if the diet can help.

A low oxalate diet can also be one aspect for the pain symptoms of vulvodynia and vaginodynia sufferers. Many doctors still consider these diseases to be "all in your head" but again, many women have found some relief on a low oxalate diet.

This too applies to patients reducing their pain and fatigue with such conditions as chronic fatigue syndrome or fibromyalgia. They have often discovered following a low oxalate diet relieves their symptoms.

Could a low oxalate help a leaky gut as well? First we need to go over exactly what a leaky gut is as this condition is fairly new in the medical community. As Marcelo Campus, MD explains in the Harvard Health Blog, "The expression "leaky gut" is getting a lot of attention in medical blogs and social media lately, but don't be surprised if your doctor does not recognize this term. Leaky gut, also called increased intestinal permeability, is somewhat new and most of the research occurs in basic sciences. However, there is growing interest to develop medications that may be used in patients to combat the effects of this problem.

Inside our bellies, we have an extensive intestinal lining covering more than 4,000 square feet of surface area. When working properly, it forms a tight barrier that controls what gets absorbed into the bloodstream. An unhealthy gut lining may have large cracks or holes, allowing partially digested food, toxins, and bugs to penetrate the tissues beneath it. This may trigger inflammation and changes in the gut flora (normal bacteria) that could lead to problems within the digestive tract and beyond. The research world is booming today with studies showing that modifications in the intestinal bacteria and inflammation may play a role in the development of several common chronic diseases.

We all have some degree of leaky gut, as this barrier is not completely impenetrable (and isn't supposed to be!). Some of us may have a genetic predisposition and may be more sensitive to changes in the digestive system, but our DNA is not the only one to blame. Modern life may actually be the main driver of gut inflammation. There is emerging evidence that the standard American diet, which is low in fiber and high in sugar and saturated fats, may initiate this process. Heavy alcohol use and stress also seem to disrupt this balance."

So, could a low oxalate diet help? It may. Speak to your physician about it. In general, you do not want to get many oxalates in your body. Like other food sensitivities, oxalate sensitivity is most commonly associated with poor gut health. If a digestive tract doesn't have enough healthy bacteria to break down oxalates, you may get chronic pain, inflammatory, allergic or autoimmune conditions. And as stated, this can be harmful and sometimes result in kidney stones on top of a leaky gut! Something you don't need! You may want to examine your oxalate intake and scale it back to see if it betters your digestion and health. Don't worry about your intake of oxalates but if nothing else is working, high oxalates just may be affecting you.

Listing of Foods with Oxalate Levels

Ok. So we all agree that spinach, yes shockingly, is a very high oxalate food and should be avoided for all those on a low oxalate diet. One cup of raw spinach averages 650 mg! But nothing ever has one answer. The scientists with the Agricultural Research Service are experimenting with oxalate concentration in spinach. They have found eight spinach varieties with less oxalate. These plants may help in lowing the levels when breeding them. But there is much work to be done. But someday, only time will tell, a breed of spinach may be OK to eat on a low oxalate diet. Research is ongoing.

While medical professionals do not agree on a definitive list of low oxalate foods, they do agree that you should limit oxalate to 40 to 50 mg per day. To test for a patient's oxalate level, a physician usually runs a urine oxalate test.

Following is a list of foods taken from the UPMC listing (University of Pittsburgh Medical Center) with some minor adjustments (additions) because it's fairly easy to follow. If you use this or another list, for example many people use the Harvard list, please make sure it's from a reputable source and is verified! Warning. There are many, many lists out there. Especially on the Internet. The best thing is get a qualified nutritionist from perhaps your doctor's recommendation if you have a question about a certain food. A good nutritionist can also help you put together a meal plan that's right for you.

So again, why is there no one list? Well, it's an upcoming field. Many foods haven't been measured for their oxalate value or they vary widely due to different researchers and methodology. This explains too why the oxalate level of foods is not yet on food labels.

This can be overwhelming. Various anecdotal stories have shown that it's very hard to follow a low oxalate diet. It is very, very restrictive and it eliminates a number of "healthy" foods. But fairly soon, you will know and stay away from high oxalate foods. At the beginning, it may be best to avoid the high oxalate foods altogether. Concentrate on the low oxalate ones. Then as you get more comfortable with what foods to choose, add the moderate oxalate foods, well, in moderation! Remember, always have calcium with high or moderate oxalate foods if you can.

It's thought nowadays that instead of eliminating certain foods from the diet completely, a better approach may be to boost your intake of calcium-rich foods. Oxalate cannot be cut out completely because most plants have some. So, if you have to have that spinach salad, have cheese on top of the greens. But before you become expert at modifying your diet to eat moderate to high oxalate foods, it's probably safer to just eliminate all high oxalate foods.

Reducing oxalate levels only by 25% compared to a patient's former diet may be the best place to start.

This slight reduction may be all that is needed. Start with this and if you see no improvement, talk to your doctor on whether you need to start measuring your oxalate levels.

HIGH OXALATE FOODS AND DRINKS

Better to avoid these completely if you can. Or, if you must have for example, raspberries, combine them with calcium, such as a yogurt or ice cream.

The following have more than 10 mg per serving. A serving size (unless noted) is 3.5 ounces (100 grams).

Drinks:

- Dark or "robust" beer
- Black tea
- Chocolate milk
- Cocoa
- Instant coffee
- Hot chocolate
- Juice made from high oxalate fruits (see below for fruits)
- Ovaltine
- Soy drinks

Dairy:

- Chocolate milk
- Soy cheese
- Soy milk
- Soy yogurt

Meat:

- None

Fats, Nuts, Seeds

- Nuts
- Nut butters
- Sesame seeds
- Tahini
- Soy nuts

Starch:

- Amaranth
- Buckwheat
- Cereal (bran or high fiber)
- Crisp bread (rye or wheat)
- Fruit cake
- Grits
- Pretzels
- Taro
- Wheat bran
- Wheat germ
- Whole wheat bread
- Whole wheat flour

Fruit:

- Blackberries
- Blueberries
- Carambola
- Concord grapes
- Currents
- Dewberries
- Elderberries

- Figs
- Fruit cocktail
- Gooseberry
- Kiwis
- Lemon peel
- Lime peel
- Orange peel
- Raspberries
- Rhubarb
- Canned strawberries
- Tamarillo
- Tangerines

Vegetables:

- Beans (baked, green, dried, kidney)
- Beets
- Beet greens
- Beet root
- Carrots
- Celery
- Chicory
- Collards
- Dandelion greens
- Eggplant
- Escarole
- Kale
- Leeks
- Okra
- Olives
- Parsley

- Peppers
- Pokeweed
- Potatoes (baked, boiled, fried)
- Rutabaga
- Spinach
- Summer squash
- Sweet potato
- Swiss chard
- Zucchini

Condiments:

- Black pepper
- Marmalade
- Soy sauce

Miscellaneous:

- Chocolate
- Parsley

Remember: ***NO CHOCOLATE ALLOWED***

MODERATE OXALATE FOODS AND DRINKS

Have no more than two or three servings of these foods per day. Moderate oxalate foods have 2 to 10 mg of oxalate per serving.

Drinks:

- Draft beer
- Carrot juice
- Brewed coffee
- Cranberry juice
- Grape juice
- Guinness draft beer
- Mate tea
- Orange juice
- Rosehip tea
- Tomato juice
- Twining's black currant tea

Dairy:

- Yogurt

Fats, nuts, seeds:

- Flaxseed
- Sunflower seeds

Fruit:

- Apples
- Applesauce
- Apricots
- Coconut

- Cranberries
- Mandarin orange
- Orange
- Fresh peaches
- Fresh pear
- Pineapples
- Purple and Damson plums
- Prunes
- Fresh strawberries

Meat:

- Liver
- Sardines

Starch:

- Bagels
- Brown rice
- Cornmeal
- Corn starch
- Corn tortilla
- Fig cookie
- Oatmeal
- Ravioli (no sauce!)
- Spaghetti in red sauce
- Sponge cake
- Cinnamon pop tart
- White bread

Vegetables:

- Artichoke
- Asparagus
- Broccoli
- Brussel spouts
- Carrots (canned)
- Corn
- Fennel
- Lettuce (iceberg and romaine)
- Lima beans
- Mustard greens
- Onions and Scallions
- Parsnip
- Canned peas
- Tomato
- Tomato soup
- Turnips
- Vegetable soup
- Watercress

Miscellaneous:

- Ginger
- Malt
- Potato chips (less than 3.5 oz.)
- Strawberry jam/preserves
- Thyme

LOW OXALATE FOODS AND DRINKS

Enjoy as many of these low oxalate foods as you like. Low oxalate foods have less than 2 mg of oxalate per serving

Drinks:
- Apple cider
- Apple juice
- Apricot nectar
- Bottled beer
- Buttermilk
- Cherry juice
- Cola
- Grapefruit juice
- Green tea
- Herbal teas
- Lemonade
- Lemon juice
- Limeade
- Lime juice
- Milk
- Oolong tea
- Pineapple juice
- Wine

Dairy:

- Cheese
- Buttermilk
- Milk

Fats, nuts, seeds:

- Butter
- Margarine
- Mayonnaise
- Salad dressing
- Vegetable oil (including olive oil)

Fruit:

- Avocados
- Bananas
- Cherries (Bing and sour)
- Grapefruit
- Grapes (green and red)
- Huckleberries
- Kumquat
- Litchi/Lychee
- Mangoes
- Melons
- Nectarines
- Papaya
- Passion fruit
- Canned peaches
- Canned pears
- Green and yellow plums
- Raisins (1/4 cup)

Meat:

- Bacon
- Beef
- Corned beef
- Fish (except sardines)

- Ham
- Lamb
- Lean meats
- Pork
- Poultry (Including eggs)
- Shellfish

Starches:

- Barley
- Cereals (corn or rice)
- Cheerios
- Chicken noodle soup
- Egg noodles
- English muffin
- Graham crackers
- White rice
- Wild rice

Vegetables:

- Cabbage
- Cauliflower
- Chives
- Cucumber
- Endive
- Kohlrabi
- Mushrooms
- Peas
- Radishes
- Water chestnut

Condiments:

- Basil
- Cinnamon
- Corn syrup
- Dijon mustard
- Dill
- Honey
- Imitation vanilla extract
- Jelly made from low oxalate fruits
- Ketchup (1 Tbsp.)
- Maple syrup
- Nutmeg
- Oregano
- Peppermint
- Sage
- Sugar
- Vinegar
- White pepper

Miscellaneous:

- Gelatin (unflavored)
- Hard candy
- Jell-O
- Lemon balm
- Lemon juice
- Lime juice

Notes on Some Favorite Foods

Remember, spinach may be healthy but it's not healthy for you! Make salads with low oxalate vegetables.

Potatoes. Sigh. These are going to be hard to give up for most people. While potatoes are not nearly as high in oxalates as sweet potatoes, they are still considered a high-oxalate food. A medium Idaho potato contains 64 milligrams of oxalate baked. A serving of half the potato contains about 32 milligrams of oxalates. Eating them with sour cream or a sprinkling of cheese will not help!

Stay away from french fries of course. Remember to stay away from potato chips too! A measly one oz. serving contains 21 mg of oxalate. Best to give these up too for the salt alone. With a low oxalate diet, it's best to reduce sodium too.

For you seed and nut lovers out there, most are high in oxalate too but you may be able to sprinkle a very small amount on your yogurt and ice cream to get your fix. But again, check with your medical provider.

Chocolate can be mixed with dairy. But brownies and cakes can be a problem. Not only for the chocolate but for the flour used. Best to find something that's on the low oxalate list rather than chocolate. And remember you are not alone. Many people have to give up all chocolate with other medical conditions!

Dairy products are good for calcium but they can be very high in salt and calories. Cheeses especially.

So be careful. And note too. While cheese is high in calcium, your skin may not benefit as much. When you eat large amounts of cheese, the ingredients and nutrients it contains may negatively affect the appearance and health of your skin.

While white flour is a medium oxalate, see if you can give up food such as white bread and bagels until you get used to being on a low oxalate diet. Note too that anything made with white flour can be trouble…such as desserts.

You don't have to worry about water being on any oxalate list like other drinks. So drink it freely! If you have a hard time drinking enough water, seltzer with natural fruit flavoring may be an option.

Meats are all safe and fish too since oxalates come from plant foods. This includes eggs which come from the poultry group not the dairy group. For vegetarians, tofu and veggie burgers are very high. Stay away from these foods. For people who are lactose intolerant, stay away from almond and soy milk, get calcium from vegetable with a moderate oxalate level such as broccoli and watercress. Speak to your medical provider about how to get more calcium too on a low oxalate diet. Fish bones are a good source if you're not a vegetarian as well such as salmon.

Anything you don't see on the list you prefer (quinoa is very popular nowadays and thought to be very high in oxalate), please ask your medical provider. The oxalate level of all foods is not reliably known as of yet. So, if you have any questions, ask and find out before you buy any food.

Other Tips for a Low Oxalate Diet

Ok, so you have your shopping list in hand and are an expert in remembering the oxalates of different foods. Remember, at the beginning just avoid the high oxalate foods and try to concentrate buying the low oxalate foods. Unless, of course, your doctor or nutritionist recommends differently due to your medical situation.

The following are some tips you might practice as well to prevent kidney stones or another health issue on a low oxalate diet.

1. Eat fewer or avoid completely high oxalate foods. Yes, this may include giving up spinach, French fries, nuts, etc. But if giving them up will make you feel healthier, try. If you can't give them up completely, remember it will always help to combine these foods with calcium.

2. Increase the amount of calcium in your diet but be very careful of taking supplements. If you're lactose intolerant, it may be tempting to take calcium supplements but you may want to reconsider. Ask your doctor if you may be getting too much calcium if you increase it in your diet and take supplements! Calcium in food and calcium pills have different effects. Calcium rich foods do not

have to come from eating dairy. Often green vegetables and some varieties of fish have as much calcium. And if you have to have a high oxalate food like spinach (not recommended!) eat it with low fat cheese. Or another thought is to have a yogurt with those fresh berries in season that you may find hard to resist. Eat and drink calcium and oxalate-rich foods together during a meal.

3. Optimize your Vitamin D levels. Vitamin D boosts calcium absorption. Optimize your Vitamin D by getting regular sun exposure or supplementing.

4. Limit Vitamin C in your diet. Large doses of Vitamin C may increase the amount of oxalate in your urine. If you are taking a supplement, it is recommended that you do not take more than 500 mg of Vitamin C daily.

5. Drink plenty of fluids. This is good advice for anyone and has been around a long time. To avoid getting kidney stones, you should aim for 10 to 12 glasses a day and at least five to six of these should be plain ole water. A tip may be to drink water at specific times of day. For example, have a large glass of water when you first wake up.

6. Eat the right amount of protein. Don't go overboard with this on a low oxalate diet. If you do, there's the risk of kidney stones and many other health problems. Limit yourself daily to four to six ounces.

7. Reduce the amount of sodium in your diet. This is true for even "healthy" people. Too much sodium causes extensive calcium loss in the urine. Limit eating processed foods such as hot dogs, sausage, canned products, convenience mixes, etc. These all have a high amount of salt. Also, there is really no need to consume deli meats on a low oxalate diet. Yes, it's harder but not necessary.

8. Don't underestimate your sweat. This comes back to the point that it's important to hydrate. The more you sweat, the less you urinate. This often allows stone-causing minerals and bond with the kidneys and urinary tract. Saunas and intensive exercise may be good for your health, but remember to hydrate to avoid the common health issue of kidney stones.

9. Taking antibiotics or having a history of digestive disease can increase the body's oxalate levels. So speak to your doctor and avoid taking antibiotics whenever possible.

Low Oxalate Help at Meals

While daunting at first, eating a low oxalate diet does not have to be bland and giving up all that you enjoy or thought was healthy.

And what about fiber? Fiber-rich foods are important and fiber is associated with many health benefits from bowel regularity to helping control your weight. But three of the best sources of fiber…dried beans, whole wheat and figs…are prohibited on a low oxalate diet. It's hard to get roughage on a low oxalate diet. You just have to know what foods are good for you. Avoid foods like spinach, and instead concentrate on cabbage, cauliflower chives, cucumber, endive, mushrooms, and peas. Cabbage is especially high in fiber. Only eat low oxalate fruits for fiber.

For breakfast, eat your calcium rich foods. You should be getting between 800 to 1,200 milligrams of calcium daily. Calcium binds with oxalate. Low or non-fat dairy products are easy to eat at this meal. Choose a cup of fortified breakfast cereal (corn, rice, or Cheerios of course!) with low-fat milk, a scrambled egg, and coffee. The Harvard list of oxalates breaks down cereals by brand name. You may now reach for cereal because it's an easy breakfast meal but may have to change your habits. Always try to have a glass of water too side by side with your coffee. This may help you drink more fluids.

What if you're lactose intolerant? Avoid substituting dairy milk with soy based products. It will be very difficult to get calcium in the diet. Many food choices to get calcium many have too much oxalate. But there is one alternative. Coconut milk. It is a popular choice with vegans as well and makes a great base for smoothies, milkshakes or as a dairy alternative in baking. But it's not perfect. Coconut milk is high in saturated fat. Check too with your doctor about using any calcium supplements. It's best to get calcium from your food.

For lunch, try to stay away from grains. All whole-wheat products should be avoided and enriched white bread should be substituted in moderation. See if a turkey sandwich with "real" turkey not deli meat is possible. Try having a cucumber salad. Fresh fruit such as apples, bananas, etc. can avoid the high-oxalate fruits.

For dinner opt for lean protein. It might be three ounces of baked fish with white rice, cooked carrots, a white dinner roll, a salad (made without spinach!) and fresh fruit. Don't add salt at the table and prepare your meal without any added salt or another high-sodium seasoning. Most vegetables contain a low or moderate amount of oxalates, but stay away from those that are considered high.

Consider spiraling vegetables, called veggie curls, instead of eating pasta. Look for packaged varieties in the supermarket or frozen versions. If you prefer to spiral your own look for the appliances now on the market. Add a sauce and some protein for a meal in minutes!

You may be able to reduce the amount of oxalate too in your vegetables by cooking them. Blanching, boiling, and sautéing vegetables will reduce the oxalate content. But remember. Cooking them too long only reduces the valuable nutrients they supply!

Snacking is often the hardest part for people on a low oxalate diet. Please learn to skip salty snacks (yes, like potato chips and even pretzels!). Choose low oxalate fruit or yogurt or gelatin instead. Crackers are considered to be OK because of the low amount of flour. Unfortunately, you have to avoid all types of chocolate and nuts. But as you feel better, you will not even want these foods as snacks.

RECIPES

Remember there is no one list for a low oxalate menu. But I have gathered some recipes here avoiding the most common high oxalate foods. And be creative too! Maybe you can tweak your own recipes by replacing some foods for others.

There are no numbers listed here because you have enough stress in your life I am sure without calculating oxalate values. And as of yet, there is no one definitive list. However, if your medical provider, doctor or nutritionist, suggests you do need to measure your milligrams of oxalate, by all means do so. It is most beneficial to be aware of the number of grams of oxalates you are eating. And consider meeting with a registered dietician to develop an eating plan for you. For most cereals are high oxalate even with milk.

For starters, these recipes can help. They focus on the foods most everyone agrees has been determined to be low oxalate. Enjoy and listen to your body! For there are no substitutions for this. Pay attention, take notes, and discover how different foods may affect YOU.

Bone Broth

This is taken from another book of mine, The Diverticulitis Handbook, I included the recipe because bone broth is an excellent source of calcium. Bone broth is very trendy and yes, you can buy it. But it is very expensive and somewhat easy to make your own! The recipe that follows was inspired by Bon Appétit Magazine. I've know people who drink the broth for breakfast too. Or it's a very healthy lunch, snack, or is a "soup" before dinner.

A real bone broth is made with bones and cuts of meat high in collagen, like marrow, knuckles, and feet. Get to know your butcher! (And now I understand why my Aunt always saved the bones after a chicken or roast!) While beef is the meat most people associate with bone broth, it can also be made with lamb, pork, chicken, veal, and more. Blanch your bones first. Cover the bones with cold water, bring to a boil, and let them cook at an aggressive simmer for 20 minutes before draining and roasting. This will help take off the unsightly grizzle or meat left on the bones.

Then roast your bones. Roasting browns and caramelizes the bones. Set the oven temperature up high to 450°. Check constantly until the bones are "done". The next step is to actually boil the bones. Do not waste the crisped brown bits on the bottom of the pan; loosen them with a little water and a metal spatula, and add those to your stockpot. Doing this adds a lot of flavor!

Ingredients:

A good bone broth doesn't need much more than the bones, onion, and garlic. This is not the time to get rid of all your "stuff" in the refrigerator!

Instructions:

Femur bones are big. Use the biggest, heaviest stockpot you've got, and fill it up with your roasted bones, plus the other ingredients based on your taste. Add just enough water to cover the bones, bring to a boil, lower the heat to a simmer, and cover. The bone-to-water ratio should be close enough that the resulting broth is intensely flavored. The bones should not be floating. This will make the bone broth taste "watered down".

Cover the pot and bring to a gentle boil. Reduce heat to a very low simmer and cook with lid slightly ajar, skimming foam and excess fat occasionally, for at least 8 hours. The more it simmers the better. Add more water if necessary.

After it simmers for quite a while, remove the pot from the heat and let cool slightly. Strain the broth using a fine-mesh sieve. Discard bones and vegetables. Let continue to cool until barely warm. Do not ever put hot broth in the refrigerator! Put into smaller containers. It will stay good for about three days, and freeze up to three months. To have smaller portions for later, put the broth in ice cube trays.

And pat yourself on the back! For you made your own bone broth!

Breakfast

Frittata with Lox and Cream Cheese – 4 servings

Ingredients: 3 whole eggs, 3 egg whites, 1 tablespoon chopped chives, ½ cup 2% milk, 1 teaspoon canola oil, ½ cup whipped cream cheese, 2 oz. diced lox.

Directions: Preheat oven to 400°. In large bowl, combine eggs, egg whites, salt, chives, and milk. Mix well. Place oil in a nonstick, ovenproof pan. Heat oil over medium heat for 30 seconds. Add egg mixture. Cook until eggs begin to set. Remove from heat. Spoon cheese evenly over mixture. Top with diced lox.

Place in oven until slightly browned. Approximately 15 to 20 minutes. Remove and cut into 4 wedges.

Mango Coconut Smoothie – 1 serving

Ingredients: ¾ cup mango, ½ medium banana, 2 tablespoons low fat coconut milk, 1/3 cup nonfat plain yogurt.

Directions: Combine all ingredients in blender and puree until smooth.

Eggs Benedict – 3 servings

Ingredients: 6 slices cooked ham, 3 toasted English muffins, 6 poached eggs, Hollandaise sauce.

Directions: Sauté ham in butter place each slice on a half of an English muffin and top each with a poached egg. Cover with Hollandaise sauce.

Ingredients for Hollandaise sauce: Makes about $\frac{3}{4}$ cup. 3 egg yolks, 1 tablespoon cold water, $\frac{1}{4}$ soft butter, pinch of salt, 2 tablespoons lemon juice.

Directions: Heat $\frac{1}{4}$ pound butter to bubbling but do not brown. Into blender put 3 egg yolks, 2 tablespoons lemon juice and pinch of salt. Blend on low and add hot butter gradually. Blend about 15 seconds until sauce is thickened and smooth.

Indian Breakfast Drink (Lassi) – 2 servings

Ingredients: 1 cup plain nonfat or low-fat yogurt, 1 cup, 1 cup apple or pineapple juice, 2 bananas, 1 to 2 teaspoons sugar or honey, ¼ teaspoon cinnamon or nutmeg, 2 ice cubes or more depending on thickness desired.

Directions: Combine all ingredients in blender and process at medium-high speed until smooth.

Coconut and Cinnamon Rice Cereal – 2 servings

Ingredients: 1 tablespoon butter, ½ cup white rice, ½ cup coconut milk, ½ cup water, 2 tablespoons sugar, ½ teaspoon cinnamon.

Directions: Cook butter in small saucepan until beginning to brown, approximately 2 to 3 minutes. Add rice to butter, cook and stir until lightly browned, about 5 minutes. Mix together coconut milk, water, sugar and cinnamon in a bowl. Gradually add to rice stirring constantly. Reduce heat to low and cover. Simmer until rice is tender about 20 minutes.

Lunch

Noodles and Cottage Cheese

This recipe has no serving size nor measurements. Adjust as needed. It's a very easy and quick dish. This was handed down from my grandmother who thought of it during the Depression. Lo and behold…it's low oxalate!

Ingredients: Egg noodles, cottage cheese (large curd is better), butter melted and browned.

Directions: Cook the noodles and drain. Mix with cottage cheese. Drizzle with melted butter.

Avocado-Watercress Ring – 6 servings

Try this "fancy lunch" to impress guests.

Ingredients: 6 ounces cream cheese, 3 cups mashed avocados, 1/3 cup lime juice, pinch of salt, 1 cup milk, 1 tablespoon unflavored gelatin, ¼ cold water, 1 bunch watercress, 1 pound shrimp (cooked, peeled, deveined), 1 cup sliced raw mushrooms, basic vinaigrette dressing.

Directions: Let cream cheese soften to room temperature. Combine mashed avocado, lime juice, and salt. Mash cheese with back of wooden spoon. Gradually blend in avocado mixture and milk. Soften the gelatin in the water 5 minutes then dissolve it over boiling water. Meanwhile, chop watercress stems into 1/8 inch lengths. Add to avocado mixture. Save leaves for garnish. Add dissolved gelatin to the avocado mixture. Mix well. Turn into oiled 6-cup ring mold. Chill. Combine shrimp and mushrooms with dressing. Chill. To serve, unmold avocado ring and fill the center with the marinated shrimp and mushrooms. Garnish with watercress.

Chicken and Cucumber Soup – 4 servings

This uses cucumber for cold weather soup rather than a salad.

Ingredients: 1 large cucumber, 1 chicken breast, skinless and boneless, 4 cups chicken stock, 2 to 4 tablespoons sherry.

Directions: Peel cucumber and cut it lengthwise into halves. Remove the seeds. Cut the chicken into thin bite size slices. Heat stock to boiling. Add cucumber and chicken. Bring back to boil. Boil for two minutes. Add sherry.

Mushroom, Endive and Watercress Salad – 2 servings

A crisp, refreshing salad that can go with a sandwich or stand alone.

Salad: ½ pound fresh mushrooms thinly sliced, 2 heads Belgian endive sliced in 1-inch-long segments, ½ bunch watercress with the tough stems removed, 2 scallions including the green tops that are coarsely chopped.

Dressing: 2 tablespoons fresh lemon juice, 1 tablespoon olive oil, pinch of salt. Combine the salad ingredients and pour dressing over salad just before serving.

Basmati Rice Salad with Peas – 3 servings

Aromatic basmati rice makes a tasty salad. Add cooked shrimp for protein.

Salad Ingredients: 2 cups water, pinch of salt, 1 cup white basmati rice, 1 cup cooked fresh peas or thawed frozen peas, ¼ cup scallions.

Dressing Ingredients: ¼ cup nonfat or low-fat plain yogurt, 2 tablespoons fresh lemon juice, 2 tablespoons olive oil, ½ teaspoon Dijon mustard, pinch of salt, white pepper to taste.

Directions: in a medium saucepan bring water and salt (if using) to a boil. Add the rice stirring until it returns to a boil. Reduce to low heat for 35 minutes and cover or until the rice is almost done. See package directions. Transfer rice to a bowl, fluff with a fork, and let cool for about 10 minutes. Meanwhile, whisk together the dressing ingredients. Add dressing to rice along with peas and scallions (and shrimp if you are using) and toss gently.

Dinner

Scallops with Lemon Oil and Papaya Relish– 4 servings

Instead of serving this over pasta, try cabbage noodles!

Ingredients: For the Scallops: 3 tablespoons olive oil, 2 tablespoons grated lemon peel, 1 pound large scallops. For the papaya relish: 1 teaspoon honey, ½ teaspoon fresh lime juice, ½ papaya cleaned and diced, 2 teaspoons chopped fresh cilantro, 1 teaspoon chopped scallions, 1 teaspoon red onion.

Directions: In a small bowl, combine olive oil and grated lemon peel. Cover and let sit overnight at room temperature. Strain mixture using a fine sieve. In a small bowl, combine honey and lime juice. Add remaining ingredients for papaya relish and mix well. Lightly spray a large sauté pan with olive oil. Sauté scallops over medium heat until cooked through, about 2 to three minutes. Do not overcook!

For the noodles: To use cabbage as a noodle replacement, peel leaves off and wash them. Slice the leaves to size "noodles" desired. Boil as you would regular noodles. If you hate the flavor of boiled cabbage, add a ½ cup of cream to the boiling water. Use leftover leaves as wraps for sandwich fillings.

Beef Tenderloin with Adobe Paste and Mashed Cauliflower – 4 servings

If you love steak and potatoes, you're gonna love this!

Ingredients: For the Adobado paste: 1 tablespoon packed brown sugar, 1 tablespoon fresh lime juice, 1 teaspoon garlic powder, 2 teaspoons olive oil, 3 tablespoons chili powder, 1 pound lean beef tenderloin cut into 4 ounce fillets.

Directions: Preheat grill or broiler. In small bowl, combine brown sugar, lime juice, garlic powder, olive oil and chili powder. Mix to a smooth paste. Spread 1 teaspoon paste on each side of beef fillets. Grill or broil to desired doneness.

For the mashed cauliflower: Cook the cauliflower for 12-15 minutes or until tender. Drain until the cauliflower is very dry, add your milk, butter, sour cream, etc. or whatever you like in mashed potatoes! Mash the cauliflower to a desired mashed potato consistency.

Chicken Scaloppini with Mushrooms – 4 Servings

Serve over white rice or this dish is delicious by itself!

Ingredients: 2 tablespoons olive oil, 4 skinless chicken breasts, 2 tablespoons diced shallots, 2 tablespoons sliced mushrooms (mixed), 4 tablespoons Marsala wine, ½ diced tomatoes, 1 tablespoon fresh tarragon, 2 cups chicken stock, pinch of salt and pepper.

Directions: Pound chicken breasts on a flat surface between sheets of wax paper until ½ inch thick. Cut each breast into 2 pieces. Heat olive oil in large sauté pan over medium heat. Sauté chicken until lightly browned. Remove chicken from pan and add shallots and mushrooms. Add wine and cook until wine has almost evaporated, 1 to 2 minutes. Add tomatoes, tarragon, chicken stock, salt. Bring to simmer and cook until sauce is reduced by half. Serve ¼ cup sauce with 2 breast pieces.

Kohlrabi Slaw

A new kind of cole slaw! Serve with meat of your choice.

Ingredients: 1 large kohlrabi, peeled, stems trimmed, grated, ¼ head purple cabbage, shredded, ½ red onion, grated, 4 tablespoons cilantro, ¼ cup raisins, ¼ cup mayonnaise, 1 tablespoon cider vinegar, 1 tablespoon sugar, 1 tablespoon salt, ¼ teaspoon white pepper.

Directions: Combine kohlrabi, cabbage, onion, cilantro, and raisins in large bowl. In small bowl, whisk together the mayonnaise, cider vinegar, sugar, salt, and white pepper. Pour dressing over slaw and mix well. Chill for several hours before serving.

Easy Savoy Cabbage with Cheese

Easy way to make this pretty vegetable to serve with your favorite meat.

Ingredients: 1 small head of Savoy cabbage, 3 tablespoons butter, pinch of sea salt.

Directions: Chop cabbage into bite sized pieces. Melt butter over medium-high heat. Once butter is melted, add cabbage and sprinkle with salt if using. Add 3 tablespoons of water. Stir to combine, cover and reduce heat to medium-low. Cook for about 20 minutes or until cabbage is very tender. If not tender yet and pan is dry, add water and continue cooking. When it's tender grate on a few shavings of hard cheese while cabbage is still hot like Parmesan or Gouda.

Desserts

Elegant Baked Apples – 4 servings

These put a twist on usual baked apples. Perfect to serve to guests!

Ingredients: ½ cup dry white wine, ¼ apple cider or apple juice, 2 tablespoons sugar, 1 tablespoon butter, 1/8 cinnamon, 4 Golden Delicious apples, ¼ cup golden raisins.

Directions: Preheat oven to 350°. In small saucepan, combine wine, apple cider or juice, sugar, butter, and cinnamon. Bring mixture to boil, stirring occasionally. Lower the temperature and simmer for 5 minutes. Peel the top third of each apple, and place apples peeled side up in baking dish. Fill cavities with raisins and pour wine mixture over the apples. Place on middle rack of oven to bake the apples, basting occasionally with wine sauce. Bake for 1 hour and 20 minutes or until apples are tender but not mushy. Serve apples warm, chilled, or room temperature with wine sauce spooned over them. And perhaps a bit of vanilla ice cream on the side?

Baked Bananas a L'Orange – 6 servings

Serve topped with whipped cream or ice cream if desired!

Ingredients: 3 firm ripe bananas, 2 teaspoons cornstarch, 2 tablespoons granulated sugar, 1/3 cup fresh orange juice, 1 tablespoon butter, 1 tablespoon brown sugar, 1/3 cup shredded coconut.

Directions: Preheat oven to 375°. Peel bananas and cut crosswise and lengthwise into halves. Arrange in a buttered baking dish. Combine cornstarch, granulated sugar and orange juice. Pour the mixture over bananas. Dot with butter and sprinkle with brown sugar and coconut. Bake for 30 minutes or until bananas are tender and sauce is slightly thick.

Old-Fashioned Rice Pudding – 6 servings

A classic and an excellent dessert!

Ingredients: 1 quart milk, ¼ cup long-grain rice, ½ cup sugar, pinch of salt, ¼ raisins (optional), 1 teaspoon vanilla extract, ¼ teaspoon nutmeg.

Directions: Preheat oven to 300°. Mix milk, rice, sugar and salt in a 6 cup buttered casserole and bake, uncovered, 2 hours, stirring the mixture every half hour. Add raisins to pudding. Add the vanilla and nutmeg and mix carefully. Bake the pudding another half hour without stirring or until rice is very tender. Serve warm or cold.

Mini Watermelon "Cakes"

Good way to eat your fruit and get water too in this simple treat!

Ingredients: 1 small watermelon, 2 cups whipped cream, Rainbow nonpareils for garnish.

Directions: Slice a small portion of the watermelon rind off. Use the flat edge to steady the watermelon on a cutting board. Slice watermelon into 2" slices. Using a 3" biscuit cutter, cut small round out of the slices. Decorate with a small dollop of whipped cream and a sprinkling of the nonpareils.

Melon Fruit Salad – 8 Servings

No high or medium oxalate berries or grapes in this colorful fruit salad!

Ingredients: 3 pounds watermelon cut into 1-inch cubes about 5 to 6 cups, 2 pounds cantaloupe, cut into 1-inch cubes about 3 to 4 cups, 2 pounds honeydew melon cut into 1-inch cubes about 3 to 4 cups, 2 tablespoons chopped fresh mint, 1 tablespoon fresh lime juice, 1 tablespoon sugar.

Directions: Place all ingredients in a large bowl and mix gently. Taste and add more lime juice or sugar as needed. Serve immediately or chill up to 4 hours before serving.

__Oatmeal Banana Cookies – 16 cookies__

Even though oatmeal is considered to be a moderate oxalate, you can have these once in a while. And have a glass of milk too. Yum…milk and cookies!

Ingredients: 2 large old bananas mashed, 1 cup of quick oatmeal.

Directions: Preheat oven to 350°. Mix two together. Add in raisins, ¼ cup, or 1 teaspoon of cinnamon. This is optional or you can add both! Bake for appoximately 15 minutes on a greased cookie sheet.

Last Word on a Low Oxalate Diet

So your doctor recommends you go on a low oxalate diet. My suggestion is don't freak out! Most people walk out thinking they can never eat spinach, chocolate, or another berry ever again. While certain foods are best avoided because of their high oxalate content, if you do give in, only do so once in a while and remember this is best in the long run for your health. Consider too that old mantra, "everything in moderation". As long as you're eating low oxalate foods 90% of the time!

Start in the beginning, and avoid all high oxalate foods. Try to buy low oxalate. After you get comfortable with this, go for the medium oxalate ones along with brand names. There are many lists on the Internet to help you with this. Make sure they are vetted! Or your wonderful dietician should be able to assist you too! Go on and enjoy the foods good for you. A low oxalate diet is not that bad at all!

Can I Ask You a Favor?

If you've enjoyed reading this book, please leave a very short positive review. I read every review personally and will take into account any feedback you may have in future writings.

Thank you so much!

Printed in Great Britain
by Amazon